Osteobiz Guide to

Fearless Marketing

Easy ideas to increase patient bookings!

Gilly Woodhouse

Sandi
Here's the key to
your marketing magic!
Love
Gilly
x xx

“In business, there is a fundamental difference between throwing money at a problem and investing in assistance.”

Gilly Woodhouse

Dedication

My special thanks must go to The Old Boy, David, who lit up my life when all around me was grey.

Also to my wonderful sons, Max and Toby, without whom this journey to Osteobiz would never have happened.

And to all my clients around the world who've demonstrated time and again that implementing this stuff leads to a fully booked diary.

Acknowledgements

Expanding a small business and adding to your team of one can be an unnerving process. However, Osteopath Jos Drew came along just as my rapid expansion was about to engulf me. Happily our clients love her calming, nurturing and supportive role as they build their own patient lists. And she shares my vision for a future where osteopathic treatment is interwoven into everyone's healthy lifestyle.

Contents

Over the years, I've had myriad ideas for small businesses, books, courses and the like. My first forays were a little shaky however.

Living on a rural Shropshire farm, I had ground-breaking ideas of creating much sought after baskets made lovingly from the strong green reeds I found in the boggy fields. There were teething problems with these. They tended to fall apart...

So moving on to the junior school classroom, I developed an amazing elixir using unusual ingredients. Well, mostly glue, powder paint and anything else squidgy that I could get my hands on. It festered in the back of the cupboard under the sink for many a long month.

Until one day it was discovered by my exceedingly annoyed teacher. He demanded to know who had made this hideously pungent and festering concoction. Pathetically, I trembled and held up my hand. I knew then that science was not for me.

Fast forward a few years and I headed to London and found a captivating place of opportunities. I began to spot niche markets and did extremely well setting up a recruitment business from scratch in the economic downturn of the early 1990's. This was purely for the world of West End commercial estate agents which I already understood very well.

Having then left to have my first son Max and then my second son, I knew that central London no longer had the magnetic pull it once did. So I began selling jewellery at house parties, often doing best when I pinned brooches on my pregnant bump and hung multiple necklaces on myself.

It was a massive shock when it transpired that little Toby was born with an incurable kidney cancer.

Life went into freefall.

Great Ormond Street Children's Hospital had to try new protocols to save his life.

Eventually, after a horrific couple of years, Toby began his slow recovery. But the chemotherapy cocktail and the radiotherapy was to eventually result in him suffering heart failure and a stroke.

But it was complicated; we were now living in Athens and for 6 years I had built up a thriving niche business there. I had noticed that so many of the ex-patriots living there were missing the delicious and convenient ready meals which you could get from M&S and Waitrose.

Being a farmer's daughter and a keen cook, I wasn't fazed by cooking in huge batches. So I created curries which were devoured with relish (haha) and shedloads of lasagnes. At Christmas I'd pull out all the stops and create mince pies by the thousand. It was exhausting, physical work in the heat but I loved building up my business and serving my community.

Toby was 12 and I was left with no option but to repatriate to London with just him in a delicate state and one suitcase with a few possessions.

The doctors said he needed an urgent heart transplant.

Great Ormond Street swung into action and soon I had the option to take him off the transplant list to see if we could encourage him to grow a bit bigger and therefore receive a slightly larger heart. He was a skinny little fellow at the time.

I began taking him to see my friend Anne Wright, a highly skilled Osteopath. Over the coming months I saw Toby begin to make a remarkable recovery in his general post-stroke state.

Simultaneously, I couldn't hope to hold down a job with a sick child to look after but I wasn't eligible for benefits. Anne suggested I did the marketing and organisation for the newly formed CPD provider, the Rollin E Becker Institute.

Talking to Osteopaths over the spread I put on for lunch, it became apparent that many struggled to find new patients and increase bookings. Before I knew it my entrepreneurial brain stepped up and I began inadvertently coaching them and sharing social media marketing ideas as well as strategies I'd used for years to grow businesses.

Early one Sunday morning the word Osteobiz floated into my mind and from there I mapped out a successful online business to help more people around the world to find the awesome hands and curious minds of Osteopaths.

Yes, it's time to be a fearless marketer and attract more patients!

This handy little book has been created for you to dip in and out of when you need bolstering up, or are looking to be inspired with fresh ideas.

Marketing works best when you are able to confidently promote yourself and the skills you offer.

In the last century, marketing for small businesses such as ours was a much simpler affair.

When you learnt your skills, there were no modules on business building strategies. Having qualified, you would have rented a room somewhere, popped a few leaflets through doors, maybe put a postcard in the local shop or an advert in the paper.

The most proactive marketing was probably putting a listing in the local phone directory or Yellow Pages (which are now defunct of course), or you might have pushed the boat out and invested in a larger square advert to get attention.

That was it.

However, with the advent of the internet, email and social media, business building couldn't be further away from what it was.

Now, you need to be rather more skilled and savvier when it comes to marketing your practice.

It's not surprising then, that having no comprehensive training in building up a busy practice, it's understandable that it can be daunting knowing where to begin.

I've noticed that what often ends up happening, is principals who aren't sure how to grow patient numbers can end up throwing money at problems to try and solve them. So they invest huge sums in 'SEO' and stick money into flickering ads on the TV in the GP's surgery. Or sometimes they'll try severely discounting their services via an online platform.

Sometimes, they'll simply sit in a deserted practice and blame the economy, the government, the holiday period or the position of the clinic. Worse still, sometimes they can think that it's their own fault that they're quiet; that they're simply not good enough. None of these things are ever true.

In my experience, once some well-crafted and targeted marketing has been consistently shared out into the community, the patient numbers begin to rise.

This book is set out as a collection of tips to help you master some easy marketing in order to increase your bookings.

First, we start with a little on confidence and mindset. It's vital that your head is in the right place and I find that's often an issue which needs tackling early on.

But let me assure you that nobody is as harsh a judge of you and your abilities than YOU! I hear some pretty terrible admonishments spoken to self.

Listen out for that and if you catch yourself being critical of your thoughts, actions or results, please reframe. The same goes for negative thinking and assumptions.

If you wouldn't say that to a family member or friend then it's not kind to speak to yourself in that way either.

It saddens me when I hear such mean self-talk when the truth is that every day you are changing lives with your magic hands, knowledge and super skills. I do believe that it is possible to act with humility as well as self-confidence.

Next, we're going to understand how to harvest great messages and words to speak back out to more potential patients.

This is crucial because unfortunately, Osteopathy is still a little-known treatment; shocking I know!

So, unlike many manual therapists, you still need to educate and inform your community about *WHY* they would book in to see you.

Once we've cracked that, getting new patients to book in for a speedy and effective treatment of their pain will be way easier.

And when we've mastered HOW to gather the information you need to market yourself effectively, we'll be looking into some basics of your website and search engine optimisation (SEO). There's so much that you can do yourself at very little or no cost.

Moving on from that, this book will explain just how vital social media marketing is to the growth of your business.

Many dislike it and don't want to engage with it at all. This is fine in the context of normal socialising however for business purposes, social media is the behemoth of our times. It certainly isn't going away any time soon, with new platforms coming to the fore all the time. So we need to harness it constructively.

You'll learn where to position yourself and how to convey your message to your potential patients in a way that hits the bullseye time and time again.

I'll repeatedly say this but educating and informing your community to understand why they would book an appointment is your fundamental cornerstone and ongoing goal.

Social media is brilliant for this and anyone who tells you that you don't need it, simply doesn't understand the power of it themselves.

Osteobiz Tip #1

Dream it.

Believe it.

Expect it.

Work at it.

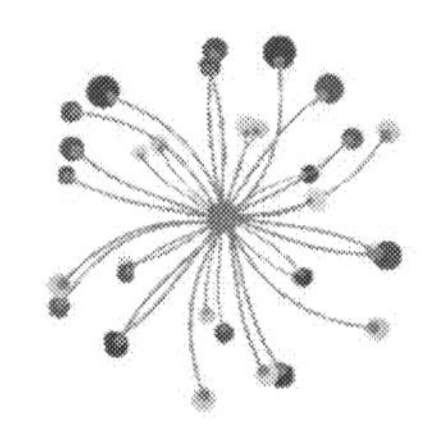

Dream it. Believe it. Expect it. Work at it. Be thankful. Rinse and repeat! What do you want to manifest? Write it down. Better still, grab a big piece of card, pens, magazines, glossies and glue. Chop out all of the images and words that resonate with you.

Sort and exclude all those that don't make you excited. Stick the rest randomly all over the card. Pop it on the wall or inside a cupboard door. Look at it every day, get excited, imagine that life. It will come – you don't need to know how, it just will if you simply take action every day.

Using these techniques, I've managed to manifest the kitchen I've always wanted, travelling extensively whilst running my business and even attracted the Old Boy to me some two years after I pasted a remarkable resemblance of him onto my vision board whilst still living in Greece...

If that's too 'infantile' for you, simply take yourself to a quiet spot, with pen and paper and write, write and write some more. Allow yourself to dream big, put some BHAGS into the mix. BHAGS?

BIG HAIRY AUDACIOUS GOALS!

I didn't know how I could possibly travel and work simultaneously, but I kept believing that the way would become obvious. And it did.

Believe in your training. Believe in your skill. Believe you are making a difference to your community. You have immense skill, knowledge and expertise. I see many worrying about things outside of their control. Or they're worrying about what their competition is doing or charging.

So, let's stand up tall and be proud of all that you do. Be proud of all the pain you have taken away from your patients this week, this month, this year! What you do all day long is amazing. The relief you bring to your patients is immense. At the end of every week pat yourself on the back for all your great work.

Osteobiz Tip #2

Be kind to yourself.

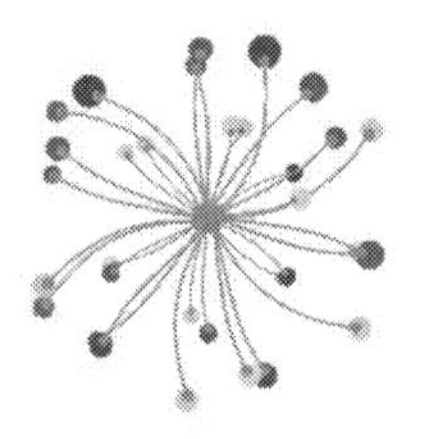

Treat yourself to a lovely notebook for your marketing; something that really draws you to it. Write down in the back of your book all the lovely things your patients have said about you. If you ever have one of those self-doubting days, read them.

Remember the grateful look in that patient's eyes, and feel again the hug or the tight handshake or the look of relief on their face.

Be kind to yourself: it's important.

What to Wear?

Some like a crisp white jacket. Some like a tunic, a polo shirt, or slacks and a t-shirt.

There's no right or wrong. If you need to wear something formal to separate your personal life from your business life, do so. If you prefer to feel comfortable as you sprint around your couch all day – do so.

Osteobiz Tip #3

Dress however you like for work but wear your Osteo outfit like armour.

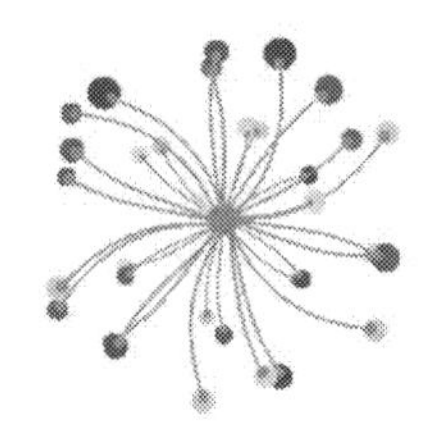

Whatever you wear, if you're sensitive to other people's energy and vibes, use it as a barrier.

No bad moods or intentions can get through your armour. Try to leave your personal worries and situations at the door and on leaving at the end of the day, do your best to leave all that patient information inside the clinic walls where it can't permeate your personal and family time and wear you down.

And if there's been too much tragedy inveigling its way into your ears this week, seek solace from an understanding colleague or friend and then let it go.

Too much emotional baggage can lead to burn out and exhaustion. Some have even thrown their clinic keys into their treatment room and walked away after feeling overwhelmed with too much stress.

Self-care is crucial; as is exercise and time for fun.

Osteobiz Tip #4

Listen carefully to your patients... their words, actions and worries are fodder for your marketing.

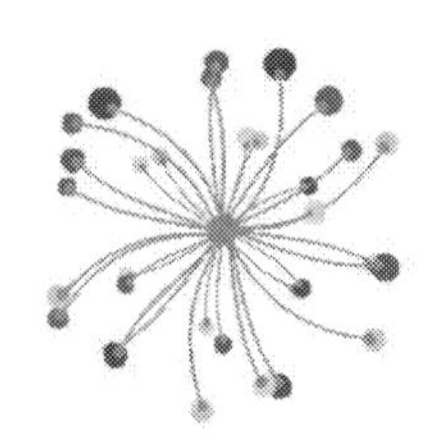

Listen Even More Carefully...

Sometimes coming up with marketing messages for social media etc. can be a nightmare. You think you should write a blog; but where do you start?

What topic should you choose and what aspect of that idea should you begin writing about?

How technical should you be? How do you pitch it?

Give up?

You're not alone!

Imagine listening to a beautiful Beethoven symphony or even a Foo Fighters' big hit. You're listening to the entirety of it, all together it's meant to be heard. But if you listen carefully, you can pick out the beat of the drum or the perfect strumming of the strings which you may not have noticed before.

This works well in clinic too! When your patient describes their symptoms, listen a little bit closer. Somewhere in that overture are a few complaints.

- What is this problem stopping them from doing?
- What can they no longer do without pain?
- What aspirations and goals could you help them with?
- What did they used to do but can't now?
- How did they used to feel and how do they feel now?
- What misconceptions do they have?

- What limitations is this problem putting on their lives?

THAT is where your marketing is: in the melody. Sing that back to more potential patients just like them and they will hear you and cheer for somebody finally understands. In that moment, they will understand why Osteopathy could help them.

Drop the Jargon

"Ooh Mabel, I've got the most dreadful musculoskeletal problem." Said NO ONE EVER!!

You may not know it, but you have the curse of knowledge! You have forgotten what it is like to not know all the correct names for all the bones, joints and muscles etc.

However, many people paid scant attention to their human biology lessons at school and probably have no idea what their sacrum is or even where to find it.

The Old Boy once fell off a low stool whilst living it up on holiday. He hilariously told everyone that he had hurt his 'coccyc' – because that's the singular, right?!

Now, the Old Boy has other strengths – such as flirting with a couple of Aussie girls in this case, so I think he got what he deserved! But now you know what you're dealing with out there in the non-Osteo world...

Osteobiz Tip #5

Reread all your content, marketing materials, website copy and social media marketing with your jargon filters on.

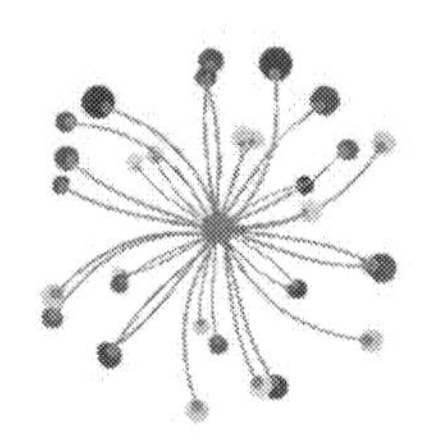

Will the Old Boy or Mabel understand what on earth you are talking about? Remember to write clearly for them – your marketing materials are not the place to impress your peers.

What can you do differently?

Be careful what you tell yourself. Success comes down to you and the stories you tell yourself.

Some practitioners don't turn up to clinic unless they have patients booked in. But what message is that sending out? You don't actually want to be busy? Some people take courses, read 'how to' blogs and ask for advice, then don't take any action. Some want change but don't make any changes!

Osteobiz Tip #6

If there are gaps in your knowledge, fill them and then take action.

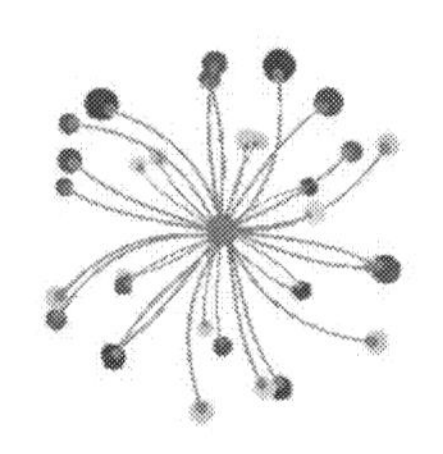

If you don't understand marketing then learn how to do it effectively. If patient numbers continue to be low or even start dropping, get some help with modern strategies.

Change is a constant. The world is progressing at a crazy pace. You can keep up but don't wait until you are such a dinosaur that it's a massive task for you.

Learn new skills. Take massive action. Implement, implement, implement. Be consistent and persistent. Success comes down to you, what stories you tell yourself and what action you take.

Excuses are dream killers. They get in your way and strangle your success and blame is a cop out.

And if you've identified that you need help but aren't sure what to do, drop me an email gilly@osteobiz.com and I'll point you in the right direction.

Trying to be 'Professional'

This is likely to get in the way of your marketing. What is 'professional' anyway? It can be a tricky word that fills people with dread. Trying to 'be something' is trying not to be yourself.

'Trying to be professional' in your marketing campaign can actually impede your ability to be successful. It can get in the way. Why? Because you end up double-guessing yourself, worrying that you may say something that might be construed as 'unprofessional' and therefore lead to inertia instead. (Not to be confused with being professional as a practitioner.)

Osteobiz Tip #1

What is really important to you? Honesty? Integrity? Value for money? Best advice? World class service?

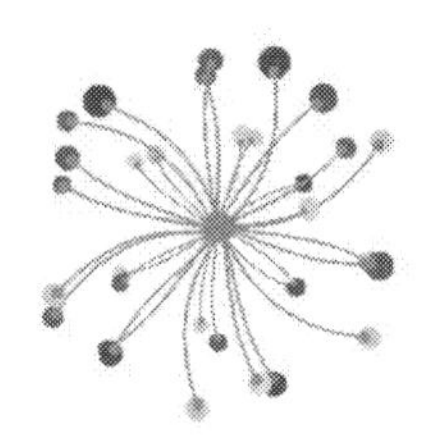

Work to those standards. Be yourself. Express yourself in your own unique way.

You will hear my clients repeating my mantra: 'people buy people', especially where you are physically interacting with another being.

If you want to grow your patient list fast, you'll need to begin by building relationships with potential patients, the fastest way to do this is by showing up and being yourself. Hang all your marketing on your core values - note them down in your book

KNOW, Like, Trust

There are not too many professions where you're working intimately with another human body.

Other examples are perhaps a dentist or an undertaker, these are also not services you're likely to pluck out of a Google search and pay for like a loaf of bread from a random bakery.

How would you go about choosing an important and, frankly, quite intimate service?

First of all you'd need to know that the service existed in your area. Then you'd need to know that they could help you with your particular problem.

Osteobiz Tip #8

Spend time, energy and a little money on great marketing which connects with your potential patients so that they understand WHY they would book to see you.

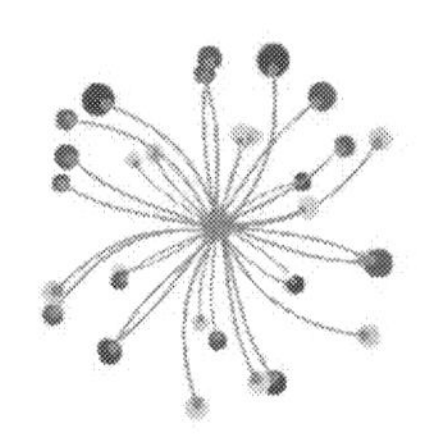

Crank up your social media content and local presence. Ensure signage is distinct and clear. Make all your marketing crystal clear and explain that you treat more than backs! Otherwise that person with an injured knee won't even consider you as a solution. Potential patients need to know you exist and they need to know how you can help them.

Know, LIKE, Trust

Have you ever gone networking and someone starts talking AT you? Have you purposefully allowed your eyes to glaze over, but they still continue with their pre-rehearsed sales pitch even though you're disengaged?

Once that point of dislike is reached, we know we are never going to that person for advice or to buy his services!

So, if you want to create long-lasting and genuine relationships with members of your community, you will need to come across as a likeable and engaging person!

Osteobiz Tip #9

Let's cut to the chase here – not everyone can like everyone but you can connect with like-minded people.

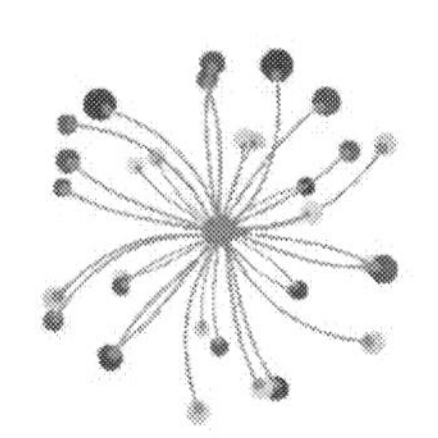

For all the people who will adore a highly successful popstar, there will be many who can't see it, can't bear them and who, quite simply, cannot see why they are popular.

And so it is for us all. Some will love us and some will loathe us. That is why being authentic is so important.

So, put on your best smile, be confident about your awesome abilities and skills and shine your amazing light on your community.

Those who like you and like what you stand for and like the service you offer will be more inclined to book to see you when they need to.

Know, Like, TRUST

Consider this: you are probably inviting your potential patients to sit with you in a small room or confined space.

They may need to divulge some personal medical history. When you examine them, they may feel nervous about what you might do, they may feel embarrassed about their bodies.

You will be treating them physically and your bodies, energies and systems are engaging with each other more than they would normally do with another person.

After that you will be expecting them to hand over payment.

And that's going to be quite a journey for many of them in the first instance. So that means they really need to trust you.

Osteobiz Tip #10

Help that unsure or nervous, next potential patient get to know, like and ultimately trust you and your skills.

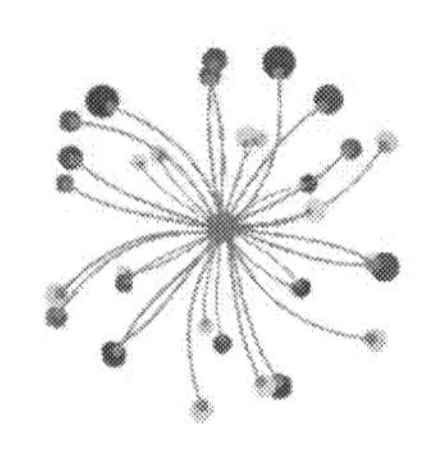

Your marketing is all about helping that nervous, potential patient get to know, like and ultimately trust you.

Because if one element is missing they are less likely to book to see you.

All your marketing needs to come together and enable that to happen.

Demonstrating your skill, experience and passion for your work will help enormously.

Word of Mouth

From 2002 to 2008, I lived in Athens, Greece and had my catering business 'Fresh Fayre'. I cooked up a storm with curries, beef wellington, Christmas mince pies and puddings and even British-style sausages.

Because my boys went to the British Embassy School, my market of ex-pats were predominantly right there in the playground every day.

My marketing strategy was simple and intuitive, just talk about it to anyone who'd listen! Very quickly word of mouth took over. During the summer I had the inevitable dip as ex-pats moved on to other postings in other countries, but those who remained would quickly befriend the new and my name would come up in passing.

Some loved to cook from scratch every day, but others sorely missed Waitrose's ready meals or a decent curry from the local takeaway.

In 2006, for the Queen's 80th birthday celebrations at the British Embassy, a huge multinational garden party was laid on for the great and the good in Athens.

There were to be food stands around the gardens offering little portions of fish and chips in newspaper cones, burgers in buns and hotdogs. I was delighted to be approached to handmake the burgers with spring onion and traditional British sausages. I remember churning out many hundreds of them and carting them up to the chef.

It was an honour to be invited to also attend and join in the celebrations. At one point a lady in a jolly dress, skipped across the lawn and with arms aloft she squealed, “Oh, you're the sausage lady! Everyone's talking about you!”

Osteobiz Tip #11

Keep talking passionately about what you do.

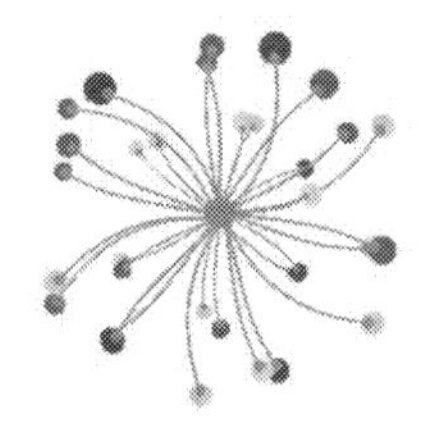

Except if you're in Australia and New Zealand, ask for testimonials from your patients. Tell them you want to help more people like them, their words are 100% more powerful than anything you could ever say.

Just remember that whilst word of mouth referrals are very valuable, it's not a strategy in itself. That's the cherry on the icing on the delicious marketing cake!

Target Markets

When I got the idea for Osteobiz one sleepy Sunday morning back in 2013, I mulled it over for a few days and wondered what it might consist of.

I talked it through with a select group of friends, family and the Old Boy. The feedback was all the same, however:

'Why are you limiting yourself to Osteopaths?'

'Why not also include Physios and Chiros?'

'Why are you niching your market so much?'

'Why don't you help more kinds of people grow their businesses and make more money?'

The thing is that I'd seen the difference that Osteopathy made to my son, Toby. But I knew that most people had no idea what Osteopaths did or even why they would visit one.

I felt quite frustrated about this, I wanted people to know how amazing Osteopathic treatment was. I wanted them to be informed so they could choose which therapy was best for them. I most definitely wanted more people to suffer less pain and take less medication.

But how could I do this?

Simple! By teaching Osteopaths how to better market themselves. By giving them the strategies they needed and by giving them better words to use in their marketing; words which I knew worked.

So, one day in the latter part of 2013 I braced myself, flipped the fear in my belly into excitement and jumped head-first.

Several years later, I have become well known and a champion for Osteopathy. I have a loyal group of followers and clients. And whilst I only ever market towards Osteopaths I also get approached by other manual therapists to work with me and that's just fine. What I teach applies to any small business.

Osteobiz Tip #12

Marketing to everyone can lead to the frustration of low bookings; be specific and that group will respond.

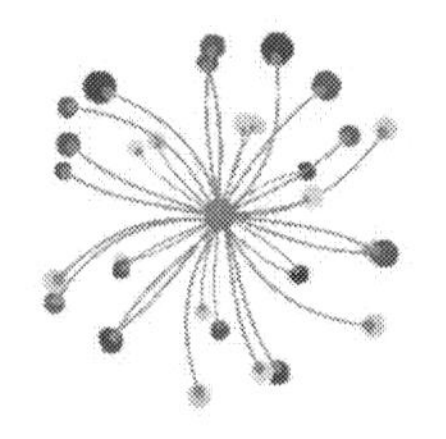

Decide on a specialism or area of interest and make your marketing very targeted to that. It may be that you love to treat the elderly, the sporty or the young. Perhaps you find that you have a special interest or a knack with something.

That can help you create very direct marketing messages, which actually land on target. Think about the words you would say to a worried mum as opposed to a competitive footballer who doesn't want to be left on the bench due to injury.

Using more specific marketing will get the attention of your target market and result in them nodding their heads in recognition. This always results in more bookings.

And don't worry, your 'bread and butter' bad backs, will still hobble in too! I would never suggest you turn anyone away or become bored treating the same problems all day long, all this means is that the effort you put into marketing actually translates into more bookings.

What is Marketing?

Back in the day I didn't really know what the difference was between marketing and selling.

But I've come to understand that marketing is all about creating and sharing relevant messages to your target market.

For example, in the UK we've seen the large German supermarket Lidl come along and cheekily target Waitrose's exact demographic. They serve up images of a lovely, happy family enjoying a superb Christmas Feast. Indeed, it's so well done that we even begin to guess that it's a Waitrose commercial.

Then the punchline comes in: 'Big on quality, Lidl on price'. And it's working! Thousands of previously loyal customers have been leaving Waitrose in their droves to cut the cost of their weekly shop.

So, if your marketing messages were just a bit better than your local competitors', how many more bookings do you think you'd get?

Osteobiz Tip #13

Do you see how important your marketing messages are? Fine tune your words and aim for the bullseye.

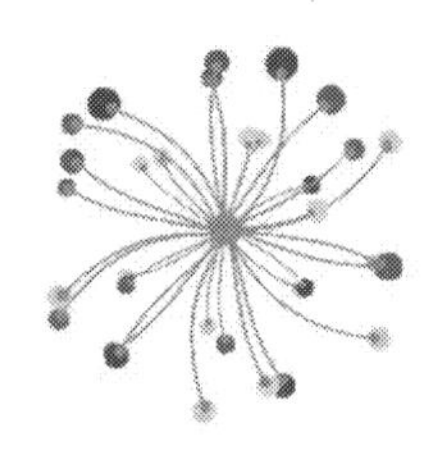

Less 'salesy' words and more information, advice and value will help people to understand why they would see you.

How to Easily Find the Best Marketing Messages

Many people struggle with what their marketing should say. For instance, their website will consist of a long, wordy and frankly dull, endlessly long page of Osteopathic studies information. It may contain lists of further CPD courses studied and all manner of other professional information; registration details etc.

But in this hectic world we inhabit, most people don't have the time or the energy to absorb all that. Generally, a person will have landed on your website via search engine results. And they're in pain.

They are looking for an answer to their question or problem.

But did you know that you have barely three seconds to capture their attention before they head back to their search results to try a different option?

Osteobiz Tip #14

Less is more when it comes to marketing! Make your words count and aim them squarely at your reader.

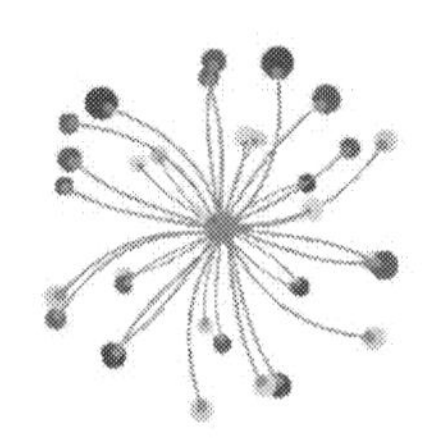

Too much text and chunky paragraphs of indigestible material is off-putting to the average person who's looking for a solution to their painful problem (as quickly as possible).

So the information they see must be easy to comprehend and get straight to the point.

If you've given the word, 'Welcome' the top billing and large font on your home page, change it! Nobody even sees that word because it's *irrelevant.*

What key message will really resonate with them? Make it concise and relevant to your audience.

Try these or adapt to suit:

- Passionate about your health?
- Helping you back to health.
- In pain? We can probably help.
- Dedicated to our community's health
- Specialising in painful problems.

What Else Should Be on My Website?

When the internet first sprang up in the '80s and businesses began using websites to market themselves, they were all rather similar and corporate looking.

But now, we have a generation who have never known a time without online information. Our online world is largely as busy as our offline world. We can search for any information and be guaranteed answers to our questions within a nanosecond.

Osteobiz Tip #15

Strip out all the dull and wordy content on your website. Make it more about your potential patient and help them understand your value.

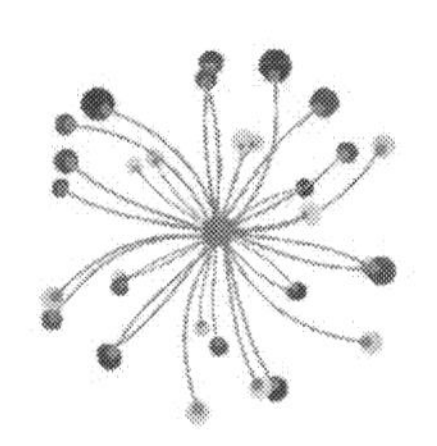

Think about why they've probably landed on your site:

- What are they looking for?
- What do they need?
- What are they not finding answers to?
- What reassurance do they need?
- What questions do they have?
- What will make you stand out from the other gazillion websites in the area?

Throw away the generic images of red pain points on bare backs, knees and hips. Instead, add local seasonal images, large pictures of each team member and a bio that demonstrates your dedication to your work.

Answer all their frequently asked questions and ditch the boring list of conditions you are 'allowed' to say you treat.

We both know that you don't treat conditions; you treat the person as a whole.

Tell them you are trained to diagnose their problems. Tell them you are qualified to refer them to a specialist or other health practitioner if need be. Tell them that helping them back to health or being pain-free is your top priority.

Genuine, honest and passionate wording is going to help more people to quickly comprehend what you do and what you stand for.

Get excited in your copywriting and allow that to ignite your potential patient's desire to trust you to help them.

And that will translate into more bookings.

What is Search Engine Optimisation?

The main search engines need to have ways to deliver up the best and most relevant answers to the questions asked by the public.

In order to make the first page of results as accurate as possible, the likes of Google need to reference every single website page they can.

They do this by ranking websites higher if they regularly find new content there. This can either be an updated page or a new blog post.

They also need to find information via keywords. These are the words that people are typing in to search bars to try and find relevant answers.

Optimising each page and blog post means that it is more likely to be found quickly and offered up as an answer.

Osteobiz Tip #16

The very best websites that enable great search engine optimisation are WordPress.

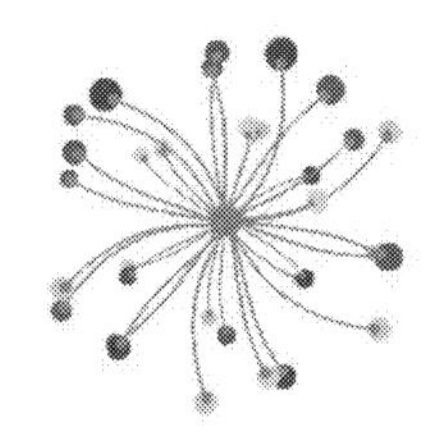

There is an abundance of WordPress styles or themes which can then be customised to suit you. Because your website is your virtual shop window, it's important not to skimp and settle for a cheap DIY-built site as it likely won't serve you well.

Simply put, that means the main search engines probably won't be able to find your website, so it may as well not exist.

Equally, you don't need a super fancy and costly website. Commission someone like Naomi Gilmour (www.happyheartonline.co.uk) to create you a beautiful and bespoke but functional website and if you're up for the challenge, she can even teach you to make your own. That way you can update it, add blog posts and make changes yourself whenever you want. If I can do it, anyone can!

How Do I Improve my Search Engine Optimisation?

SEO used to be a big mystery to most of us and something only to be handled by the experts. Huge sums were paid to 'get you up the ratings' with many promising first page results.

But these days it's perfectly easy for your web designer to do the main optimisation and for you to maintain and improve on this as you go.

Osteobiz Tip #17

Add the plug-in 'Yoast' to your WordPress website

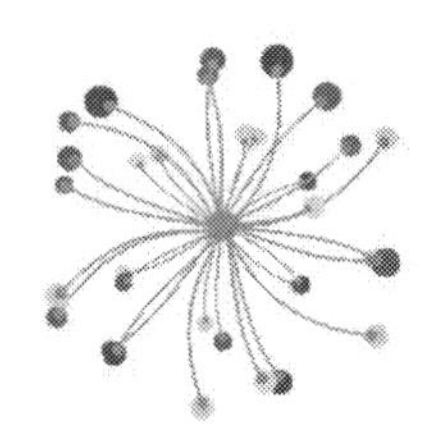

This will automatically add a section at the bottom of each webpage and each blog post.

Let's say you wanted to add a new blog post on headaches. Obviously, this word needs to appear in the title of the post, it will then automatically appear in the URL (Uniform Resource Locator) for that page. Ensure that this keyword appears in the first sentence of your post, preferably the first word you use if that makes grammatical sense.

It's best if you use a relevant image for each post to make it more interesting. Use your own where possible. When you upload it via your 'add media' button, you will see there is information about the image size etc to the right of the image. Where you see 'alt tag' (alternative tag) also add your keyword here. Did you know that Google is blind? Therefore, it cannot see images but can only bring them into a search if it can 'read' what the image relates to.

It's a good idea to break your 300 – 500 word blog up with a couple of headings (or Heading 2 as it will be called in your font size selection area). So, your keyword needs to be part of these sub-headings.

Mention the keyword as part of the main text two or three times to clarify the topic too.

Beneath the text box space, Yoast will have added a space for your keyword so that it can assess how well you have optimised your post. It works on a traffic light system and so always strive for green!

Below that is the meta description box, which will have used the first 300 characters of the text you have just uploaded to the page. However, this could mean that it's not entirely clear what the piece is about. It's often wiser to rewrite this description in the box and make it obvious what the topic is and what the reader will find out. With our example you could begin with, *'Find out why headaches begin, what triggers them and what you can do to prevent them'*.

Something similar to this will likely encourage a person to stop and read, rather than a seemingly random sentence which gets cut off at a strange point. Yoast will assess how well you've optimised your article and give you hints as to how to make improvements.

Why would you bother to do this? Because it may be that someone searching for answers about their headache problem may find your blog post, rather than a website page, and decide to find out if you can help them after reading it and seeing that it is your area of interest.

Osteobiz Tip #18

Blogs are a great way to educate and inform your potential patients and help them understand how you can help

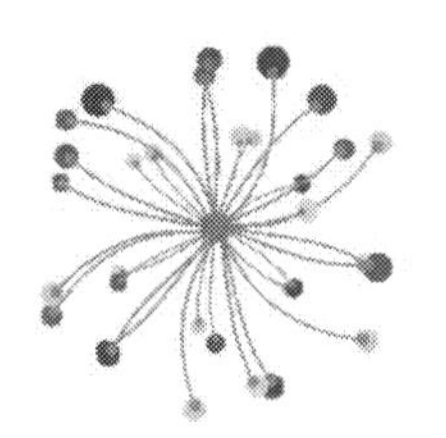

What is a Blog Post?

Blog posts are a collection of mini articles on one of the pages of your website. It's like your library of advice and information. It can be an excellent resource for your patients. Within the blog page you can create blog posts. You need to add a new and separate post each time; each one on a different subject.

It's a good idea to classify them into topics such as health, fitness, pregnancy etc. That way a visitor to your site could search for 'pregnancy' and find all the blogs relating to that subject.

They are a great way to educate and inform on various topics in which you have expertise. They also allow you to explain different concepts such as staying healthy or monitoring mobility as we age. When you know your target audience you can tailor them exactly to suit. For instance, if you were addressing an audience of doctors, you could happily use medical terminology, reference your statements, add common abbreviations and jargon and they would still understand.

However, your target market is usually the general public who may not know their cranium from their coccyx!

How Long Should a Blog Be and Should I Reference the Content?

Blogs are mini articles and are written firstly on your website and are great content for your social media. It's a good idea to decide upon the frequency of your blogs and stick to that.

Once again this is content which will build up your marketing resources over time and can be reposted multiple times. Indeed, I still have a couple of blogs, about my journey and Toby's and health issues, being reposted to social media regularly. You'd be amazed how many Osteos I've been connected to for several years who still haven't seen them and don't know why I'm so passionate about Osteopathy. It can come as quite a surprise!

Never worry about posting your blogs too many times because, even if it was read last year, a person may reread it and gather more from it a second time.

Generally speaking, the optimum size for a blog and one that's not too arduous for you to write is around 300-500 words. That way you can break down a topic, such as sports injuries, into many blogs. You could blog about typical injuries, when to apply hot or cold packs, how to warm up effectively etc. There could be advice about injury prevention, improving range of motion, when to seek your help etc.

I don't recommend referencing your blogs for two reasons:

- Referencing distracts from the flow of the piece and if they are live links you may be sending your potential patients off to another site!
- The point of your blog is to give your expert advice and encourage potential patients to book in to see you if they realise they need help.

Referencing blog posts on your own website is recognising others as the experts rather than yourself and that isn't helpful.

Furthermore, I urge you not to waste your valuable time doing extra research! You already know all you need to know about your specialist subject. Think about what kinds of tips and advice you share with patients every day. Jot those ideas down and you'll never be short of a blog topic.

Osteobiz Tip #19

Keep your blogs short and succinct.

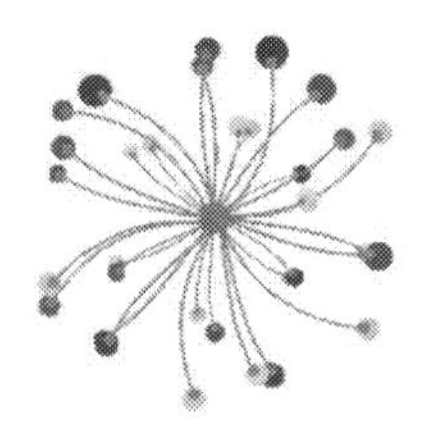

Sentences should be concise and not overly wordy. Break up the text with frequent paragraphs, headings and images if appropriate.

Use bullet points to help speed readers absorb information fast.

As previously mentioned, references are not required as that is a distraction to your reader and links to other websites do not serve you! If necessary, you could say '*recent articles in the papers about overuse of anti-inflammatories might be confusing. Here's my advice*' or '*The recent research on obesity suggests X. If this worries you, here are 3 tips for you to try*'.

Short, sharp and informative works best, saves you time and hits the spot.

Your posts also enable you to stand out as an expert in your field. This helps you attract more patient bookings when they can see that you will readily understand them and their issues.

There's nothing worse than seeing that the last blog post on a website was some time last year. It looks like the website isn't cared for and that the owner may not care either.

Decide on the frequency of posting which suits you best - be that weekly, fortnightly, monthly and diarise dates. If you can write something topical, seasonal or for a World or National Day, for Osteoporosis, for example, even better.

Is a Blog Post a One Trick Pony?

The short answer is no! You can write many posts on the same topic. Simply come at it from a different angle.

Osteobiz Tip #20

Blog topics - think about your perfect patient and what they frequently ask you.

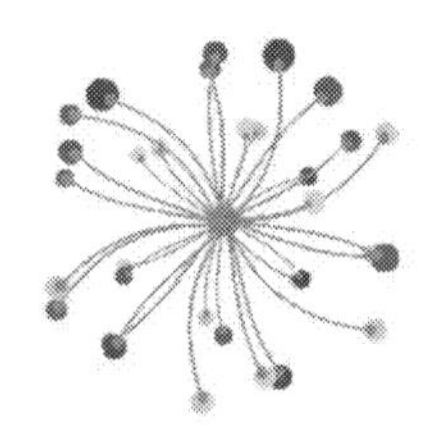

If you have an interest in treating sporty people you could write a range of blogs on key exercises for footballers, tennis players and snowboarders etc.

These blogs can be posted over and over again on social media. Many people won't see it the first time you post it and even if they do, they may take away more information and tips on a second reading, so don't worry about repeating yourself!

You can also scan the article for stand-alone sentences which can make a small social media post with a link back to the blog. Or you could cut and paste the whole blog onto a Facebook post and add an appropriate image. Take the key theme or salient points and make some memes (images with text) for your social media.

You could turn it into a podcast or use the topic to create a video.

A new or existing blog post is a handy piece of content for your regular newsletter too.

Why Do I Need A Newsletter?

An email newsletter is a great way to keep in touch with existing patients. After all the time and energy you've put into attracting them, it makes sense to occasionally keep in touch with them after a few sessions of treatment have ended.

If you're keen to continue caring for your patients' welfare, you'll be keen to share topical and seasonal information with them.

Osteobiz Tip #21

A regular newsletter to your patient list helps to remind them that you're there when they need you.

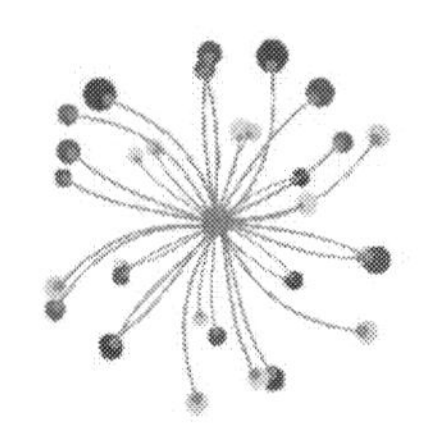

Imagine your perfect patients sitting before you and share with them the key points which will be of interest and use to them.

Reassure them, educate them and weave in your expert knowledge. Even mention typical issues or problems and responses to treatment.

Write freely for the first draft, making two or three key points. You can edit it and tighten up the structure afterwards.

Use headings or questions to break up the text, keep the paragraphs neat and sentences short.

Don't forget a great image to complete your newsletter, and either publish it or be super organised and schedule it to go out on time for the next due date.

Osteobiz Tip #22

Decide on the frequency of your newsletter and diarise.

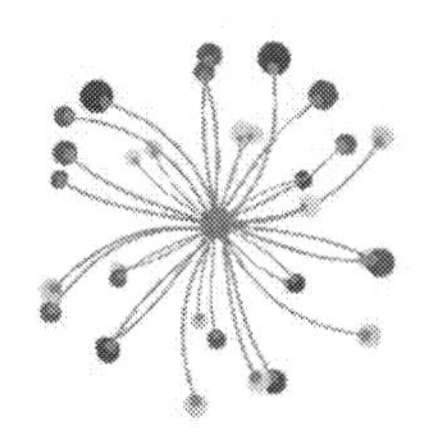

Consistency is key here. Include two or three types of information such as a taster of your latest blog and a link back to that exact item. Put the URL link behind the words, *'find out more here'*, for example.

You can also add images with seasonal tips to the mix and for seasonal holidays or for your own time off, give them closing and opening dates. Watch your bookings rise as they rush to catch you before the break!

Remember that fewer people will bother to open an email with an uninspiring title such as *'April Newsletter'* but would be curious to find out about *'3 Mistakes Runners Should Avoid'*.

NB: Do make sure that each and every patient has signed an agreement to receive newsletters from you.

Can I Send e-newsletters From My Hotmail Account?

With Data Protection being given higher precedence recently, it is vital to respect the wishes of patients past, present or future, to decide if they wish to receive your newsletters or promotional information.

There are key differences between a generic email and an email campaign system. A proper system such as Mailchimp allows you to divide up your patients into different lists, see who has opened each newsletter and who has clicked on a link to your blog post, for example.

However, the most important difference is that if a newsletter recipient no longer wants to hear from you, they can unsubscribe from your list. Now this is mandatory.

At first, if someone unsubscribes from your list you can feel rejected and take it personally. But, these days, most of us have far too many emails flooding our inboxes all day long; we simply cannot read every one.

It is, therefore, vital that your patients can unsubscribe from your newsletter list. They may simply have moved away or no longer wish to hear from you. But the option must be theirs.

Osteobiz Tip #23

Newsletters are a great way to keep in contact with your previous patients and share valuable knowledge.

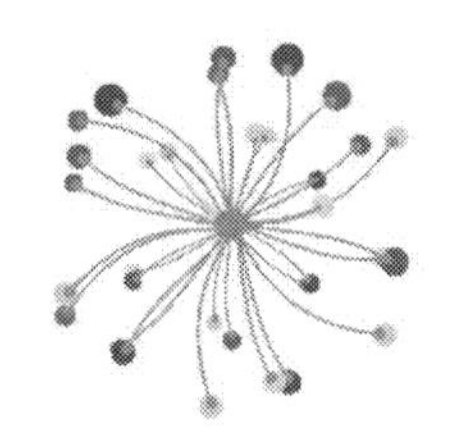

If you haven't got an e-newsletter system in place, make this a priority.

A well-crafted newsletter allows you to keep your patients up to date with any Practice news or local news. It also allows you to share more information which they may find helpful. Most importantly, it is the nudge to remind them not to put up with niggling pain.

You might be surprised at how many of us do, without thinking it could potentially be treatable. In the past, I have even put up with a painful hip which I squarely blamed on my two boys for sitting on my hips as chunky toddlers. Every morning, as I got out of bed, I did a weird sort of chicken dance with flapping wings for a couple of minutes as I tried to settle the soreness.

After months of this, it one day occurred to me that perhaps Osteopathy could help and of course it did sort out my problem in no time at all.

But I bet you I'm not the only one! An occasional newsletter simply reminds us that you're there and ready to help with niggling aches and pains.

How Can I Avoid Burn Out?

Over the years, I've heard of many Osteopaths who have worked so hard that they burn out. Some have packed in too many patients each week, some will take extra bookings to accommodate patients and let it eat into their family time or downtime, some will juggle family responsibilities with a demanding patient list and yet more will work up to seven days a week because of high demand.

It can even be that the level of emotional dependence on an Osteopath can exhaust them. They can become ill with stress-related problems or chronic fatigue-type symptoms.

Avoiding burn out is all about self-care. For many Osteopaths this isn't a high priority as there's a natural tendency to put patients first.

Osteobiz Tip #24

Grab your annual diary and plot regular time off work.

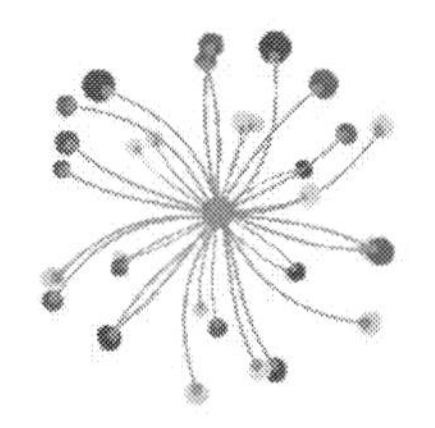

Block off chunks of time throughout the year and give yourself a few long weekends too so that you can kick back or take a mini trip somewhere lovely or veg out and get a massage!

Add in any advanced dates you have for CPD courses or conferences.

Next, clear one or two hours per week for marketing activities. If you're the Principal, strike out sacrosanct time for accounting, admin or networking events. Stick to those boundaries so that you have time to get these jobs done rather than them ending up being done late at night.

Build in emergency appointment times so that if they're not taken you go home earlier, take some exercise or run an errand.

Ensure you take proper breaks in your day. If you work a long day, factor in an extra-long lunch to rest, exercise and prepare for the afternoon.

If you're largely at full capacity ensure that all admin and accounting tasks are delegated to a virtual assistant, for example, or employ a cleaner to ensure that your practice is spotless, without added pressure on yourself.

The cost to employ help is very low in comparison to your hourly rate and your health!

None of us can do our best work from a place of lack or feeling utterly knackered!

How Can I Feel More Confident In Myself?

One of the most likeable aspects of your average Osteopath is their humility and decency.

But some practitioners can feel unsure of themselves or lack confidence.

Confidence rather than arrogance, is a wonderful trait and something we want to feel from any professional we consult.

A confidence issue is readily picked up by patients and can lead to them feeling unsure themselves!

The critical thing to remember is that low

Usually this is simply not the case!

Osteobiz Tip #25

Remember...

1. You are incredibly skilled and knowledgeable.
2. You are highly trained.
3. Re-read all your testimonials and remember the difference you make to your patients' lives.

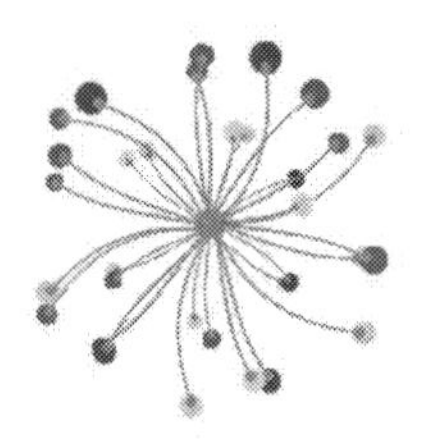

How Can I Get Seen Online?

These days, our online worlds are just as busy as our offline worlds.

The vast majority of us keep our phones and devices near us, we check what is going on in our social media newsfeeds frequently. We book tickets and restaurant tables online, we check the weather and news online. We can even check our bank balances or pay our taxes online.

The online world is now such a hectic and crazy place that to be noticed you have to be a little different.

I recently consulted my branding expert, Vicki Nicolson at www.vickinicolson.com and asked her to review my branding and especially how I use it on my website.

Expecting her to suggest some changes I waited for her call.

Vicki came back with the big thumbs up. She told me that, in theory, the colours of red, blue and a weird mustard colour shouldn't work but they did! She thought that the overall impression of my branding was punchy, different and that there was absolutely nothing fundamentally she would do to change it.

Hence my recent rebrand has been more of a 'growing up' of Osteobiz and what it stands for. I have evolved over the years and now my branding reflects that rather better than it did.

What was apparent from our initial discussion however, was that I had managed to select colours and fonts which made me stand out online. These factors meant that I would be more likely to be remembered and easily recognised as me and Osteobiz no matter whether this was on my website or social media platforms.

Osteobiz Tip #26

Branding colours and fonts need to help you stand out from the crowd.

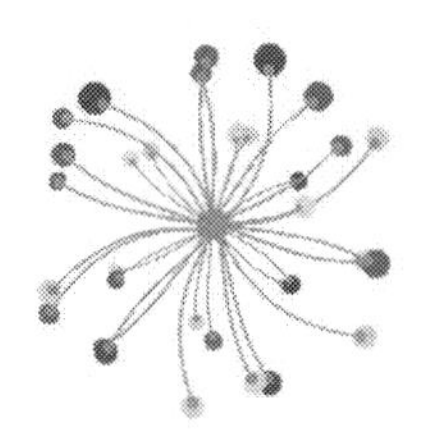

The number one way to be seen online is to ensure your branding colours and fonts are always consistent across all platforms online.

You need to know your hex codes for your colours and the names of your fonts. Use these across your social media headers and content. They need to be used throughout your website as well as on all signage, letterheads, leaflets and business cards.

Search online for a hex code generator from your logo image so you can get an accurate colour identifier.

What Exactly Is Branding?

Branding is a style for your business. It's the confident use of the exact same colours and fonts as well as your style of presentation which helps you to be recognised and remembered.

I used to work for a local Estate Agent on Saturdays. Well, it kept me out of mischief while the Old Boy played golf!

Having banged on all week about the importance of branding it used to drive me insane in the office on a Saturday.

There were leaflets using a dark chocolate colour next to business cards with a reddish hue. Then the signage outside was rather more russet. And the website brown was more the colour of effluent!

It was such a mess it was confusing. I could never tell which colour was the true one. Indeed, it looked as though a colour-blind team member guessed at it each time.

If I felt confused, imagine how it left others feeling? It gave off mixed messages and it looked sloppy.

Small wonder then that their business was in decline. As luck would have it, I jumped ship just before my branch office closed down.

Osteobiz Tip #27

Create a branding style which personifies you and the clinic.

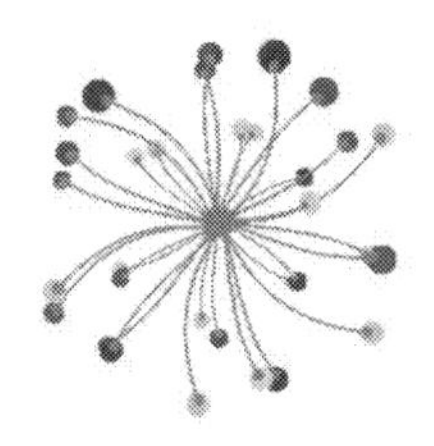

Now a business isn't going to fail purely because of inconsistent, dull or poor branding.

However, with the online world being so very busy, you need to be instantly recognised from all the options which may pop up in a search engine result.

You might imagine that I look at many hundreds of online sites and social media pages I look. Some are confused and disparate.

Check that you know your colours, fonts and type of style you use in social media post and don't deviate!

Three to five colours work well – originally, I stuck with just three as it was easier to manage.

For your fonts you will need a headline style, which is a high impact one; a fancier more interesting one for subheadings and artwork and an easily readable simple font for general text. There's nothing worse than website fonts that are so fancy you can't read them on a laptop let alone a phone screen.

How Can I Best Use Social Media For Marketing?

This is a huge and wide-ranging topic so let's start with the basics.

First of all, social media can be a vast time drain and before you know it you can be drawn into back to back crazy cat videos!

Try to separate your own social media time from your business marketing social media time. Not easy I know, but with your Osteobiz hat on you can concentrate on what your marketing strategy is rather than ending up being a bit random!

Osteobiz Tip #28

Concentrate on showing up where you know your potential patients are.

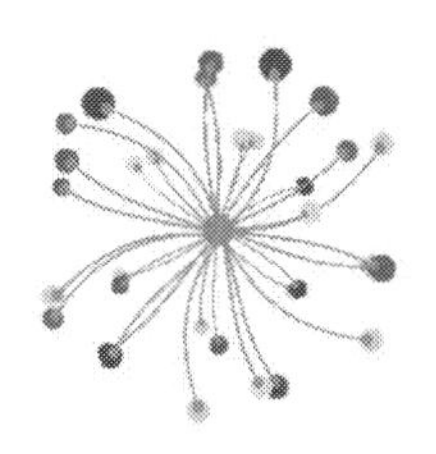

Talk to your patients for at least a week and find out where they hang out online. That's where you concentrate your time, and nowhere else.

A couple of platforms probably works best if you want it to bring more bookings and not drain you of all your energy!

Do I really need to be on Facebook?

There are currently around 3 billion users on Facebook – equivalent to nearly twice the entire population of China. That's a lot of potential patients...

Facebook has cleverly created a business platform within its framework which allows us to connect with our audience. At the time of writing there is no other social media platform which is quite so well-constructed.

Osteobiz Tip #29

Facebook is a fast way to connect with your community.

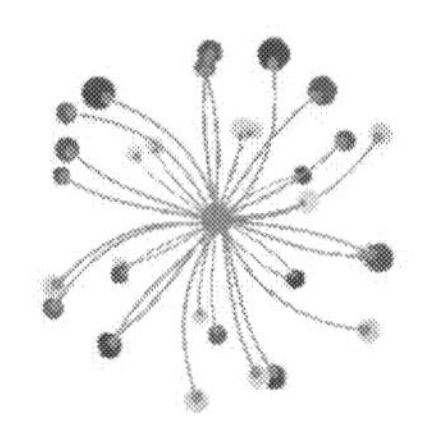

I'm all in favour of free marketing and with most of your target market being on Facebook, I'd say you'd be wise to have a presence on Facebook.

Be aware that many people use the search feature at the top of the Facebook Home Page to find what they're looking for, so it makes sense to be present!

Should I Just Have a Personal Profile And Another One For My Website?

Facebook keeps a close eye on what's happening on their platform. They have strict codes of conduct and act swiftly if they believe their rules are being broken.

Their top priority is for Facebook to be a place to find out what your friends and family are doing and talking about. In particular, they encourage interaction, connection and a deepening of communication and relationships. How many of us have hooked up with old school pals there or friends we've lost touch with over the years?

With this in mind they have two very different types of pages: the Personal Profile which you use as a personal page for yourself and the Business Page; which is only to be used for that purpose.

Osteobiz Tip #30

Your Facebook business page is the showcase of your talents.

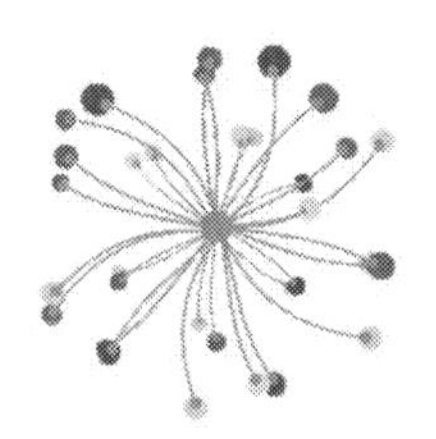

Double check that your business page is built off the back of your personal profile.

Using a personal 'professional' profile page is self-defeating for two key reasons:

1. You won't have the functionality and insights about your page followers and this is very important information.
2. You risk having both your pages shut down because you've flouted the rules.

Remember that the distinct difference between a Personal Profile and a Business Page is that you have 'friends' and your Osteobiz page has 'likes' and 'followers'.

I suggest you check right now that you've got this correct before you do anything else!

What are Facebook insights?

It's worth periodically checking out your insights for further information about the general demographic of the people who like your page.

These insights will give you details about the key age groups of your likers. It will tell you where they are based, and the proportion of male to female, etc.

Osteobiz Tip #31

Facebook business page - check your demographics.

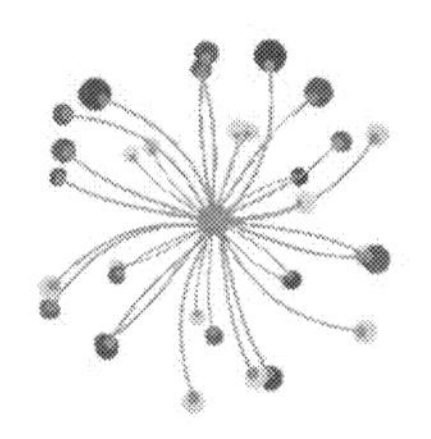

Angle your marketing towards the 2 key demographic areas if you are not already.

If the majority of your followers are 25-45 and women, you need to post items relevant to them, for example. Their areas of concern about health and fitness will be quite different from men in the 45-65 age bracket.

If you haven't got a well-defined target market this may well be a place to begin.

I've Opened A Facebook Business Page, Now What?

To start with, Business pages have evolved to cover every kind of business imaginable. It's worth spending a couple of hours on it if that's what it takes to set it up correctly.

The tabs down the left hand side of your page can be dealt with one at a time so that all your relevant information is accurately added.

Osteobiz Tip #32

It's a good idea to optimise your Facebook business page.

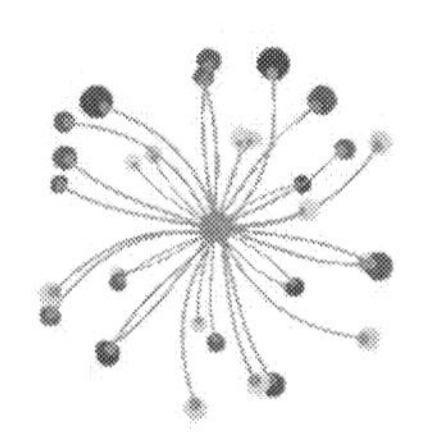

I highly recommend that you complete every section of your business page so that when a potential patient looks around, they will find everything they want.

Ensure you add your address; so the map is available for new patients, your opening hours and contact details etc.

Over on the right is an 'About Me' section. This is your opportunity to showcase yourself and your practice. Equally, it needs to be more about your patients and what you want for them. This is a chance for you to talk about your goals for your patients and why you want to help them etc.

Can I Just Upload My Logo For the Profile & Cover Image?

Facebook is a highly visual platform. Its purpose is all about getting connection and engagement with people who might need your help.

It is highly effective as a marketing tool and a little time and energy are all that's needed to make it work well for your business. However, that time and energy needs to be used cleverly to maximise the number of people who see your posts.

The majority of people will see your posts in their newsfeed mixed in with recent posts from friends and family. Some will want to know more about you and what you do and they will visit your entire page. That's why everything needs to be attractive, compelling and interesting.

There is nothing quite as dull and uninspiring as a logo being overused on social media!

Osteobiz Tip #33

Facebook business page – get your first impressions right.

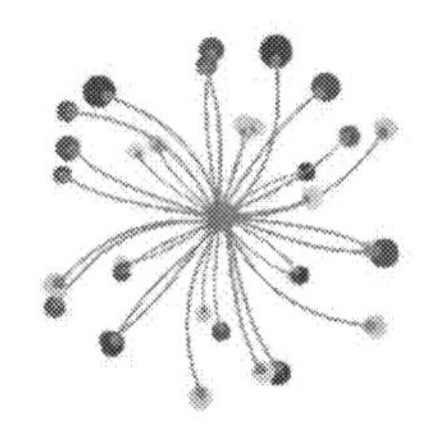

In a similar way to your website, your Facebook Page is the online shopfront representing you, your values and your service.

Therefore, first impressions count very highly. Go and take a look at your Osteobiz page; who is looking back at you? Is it you? Or is it an impersonal logo? Your logo doesn't use its hands on patients; you do! It can feel uncomfortable to put yourself out there, I know. However, I will be repeating this many times – 'people buy people' – not logos, websites or social media pages.

These things represent us, our values and our services but it is crucial that we show ourselves to our potential clients so they get a feel and flavour of our character and what we stand for.

If you haven't already, take a look at my Facebook Page Osteobiz; see how my face, personality and dedication for you and your work shines out. That is one of the ways I've taken my business from a vague idea to a successful worldwide enterprise.

To get the best results from social media marketing you must put your stamp on it.

Therefore, even if your picture is only taken with a phone, do get it uploaded today. Make it close up and smiley. As you will know, looking into another's eyes and reading their face is the first way we decide if we like someone.

Miss that step out and you've probably missed out on the opportunity to engage with a new patient.

Ok, I've got My Social Media Platforms Sorted, How Do I Sound Professional?

The first rule of social media is that it is social!

Many Osteopaths get hung up about being 'professional' in their social media marketing. But what does that mean? Does it mean impersonal, cold, characterless and boring?

Attempting to be 'professional' on social media is defeating the object. I'm not suggesting that you do or say things that contravene your professional code of conduct or conflict with the advertising standards either.

I'm talking about relaxing somewhat with your potential patients in the same way you would be face to face in clinic.

Sometimes when we put things out there via the internet it can feel that we're broadcasting to the world. That can feel very unnerving. Worse than that, it can feel like we're exposing ourselves to criticism, ridicule or judgement.

Osteobiz Tip #34

Having gone through this process myself, I have realised:

- Not everyone is going to like you.
- Not everyone will agree with Osteopathic treatment.
- Not everyone will agree with what you say.

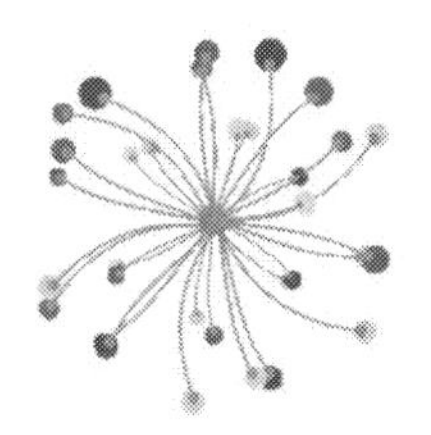

So you might as well stand up, be yourself, talk about what you believe to be true and share your passion for your work.

Those who love what you say and resonate with your values and objectives for their health will book to see you.

Those who don't will likely never become a patient.

And that is the same for all of us in business.

How Do I Get My Tone Right? I'm Worried I Might Offend?

I get asked this quite often and it largely follows on from the last question.

Once again, it's important that your marketing sounds just like the real you; remember I said before that people buy people?

I regularly run workshops and lectures. I'm a prolific blog writer and am highly active on my social media platforms. I should add, that is how I've built up a thriving business.

Getting the tone right in all of this can sometimes feel tricky. But if you can convey how you care, what you're passionate about and how you help, you'll be developing those all important relationships.

I've been doing exactly this for many years now.

The interesting feedback from most of my personal interactions with Osteos is that I turn out to be exactly who they thought I would be from the tone of my writing.

For me, that is very reassuring and here is why. If I had tried to write my social media content in a way I thought my audience would want it, it would come across as fake or false. For instance, if I wrote in a light-hearted and humorous manner but when you met me I was dull and boring, your instincts would warn you not to trust me.

Osteobiz Tip #35

Create content that reflects YOU.

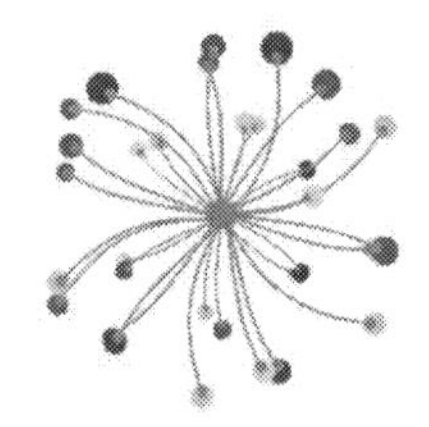

Whether your general manner is funny, passionate, concerned, charming, caring, warm, a bit direct or blunt, you might as well be yourself.

It's better to show your character than tone down everything so that you came across as dull, miserable or devoid of personality. Shine your light out there and shine it brightly!

What is Social Media Content?

'Content' is the generic name for the collection of posts you put on your business media pages.

There are many kinds of content and it's important to mix it up so that your page as a whole is engaging and interesting to many kinds of people.

Some people love to read an interesting article because they are thoughtful. Some like to watch videos because they're commuting to work and want to be entertained. Yet others will love short tips and visual messages because their attention span is... ooh look a butterfly!

The following are general types of content:

- Blogs
- Infographics
- Testimonials (not in Australia)
- Memes
- Videos

- Case-Studies
- Tips
- Lives
- Local news
- Advice
- Inspirational Quotes
- Photos

Osteobiz Tip #36

Mix up your content so all kinds of people will find something of interest to them.

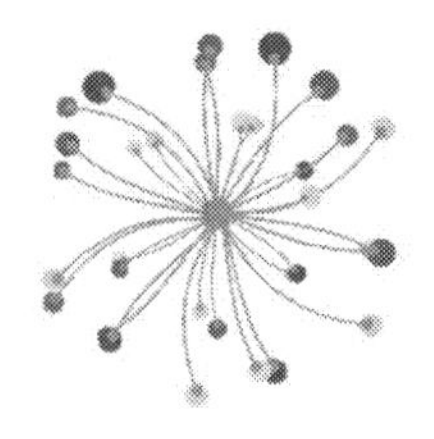

Go and check out your social media platforms; is there a good mix of content types?

I've seen business pages (even business coaches!) where the type of posts are only a long line of blog links or repetitive testimonials and nothing else! And others where they are only urging people to 'book now, book now!' or there's only plain text posts with no images to catch the eye.

Remember that people are generally whizzing through their newsfeed on their phones, scrolling until something catches their eye. What will attract the attention of your target audience?

What Sort Of Mistakes Should We Avoid?

I spend a huge amount of time looking at Osteopaths' social media pages. Here are the key mistakes/issues I spot:

- Not posting for weeks or even months at a time.
- Mostly only posting text with no images.
- Sharing other people's content.
- Only pressing for bookings.
- Forgetting to serve their followers first and sell second.
- Talking to people in the plural.
- Having incomplete information e.g. no website link.

- Being so anonymous that I can't even tell if the Osteo is male or female or what their name is.
- No original content.
- Sending potential patients to media websites.
- Failing to help us understand why we should book.

Osteobiz Tip #37

Start with a strategy.

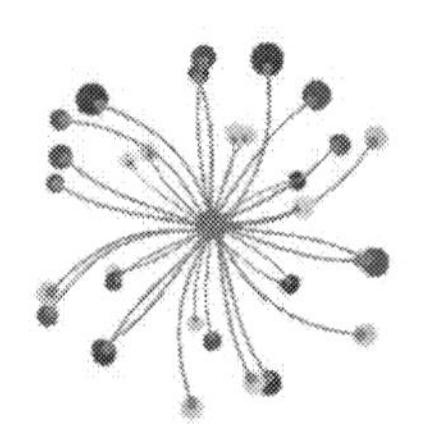

Begin with a strategy rather than pushing random stuff at your followers and hoping some of it will stick.

Answer these questions to define yours:

- WHO am I trying to attract more of (be specific)?
- WHAT do they need to know to help them with their goals/pain/condition?
- HOW does Osteopathy benefit them?
- WHY would treatment help them?
- WHEN should they seek treatment?

What if I'm Still Struggling With Ideas For Social Media?

This is actually a very common problem. It's really a kind of content constipation! This comes about mainly because of overthinking and being concerned about peer judgement.

Let's start with the latter. Your social media marketing – or any other kind – is nothing to do with your peers! They are not your target market. The people reading your posts are nowhere near as educated in healthcare as you are. If they haven't yet found Osteopathy, it's likely that they are conditioned to stick with standard medical and drug-based healthcare.

Your job therefore, is to simplify your messages so that they hit the target accurately. Indeed, the more basic the message, the better! Helping ordinary people in pain to understand that they have other options, such as Osteopathy, is all you have to do.

Moving on to procrastination and overthinking – this is likely to be you getting in your own way. Let's be clear here, shall we? You don't need to do any more research, any more CPD or any more courses in order to put out an effective message.

What you do need to thoroughly understand is how your potential patients are feeling, how their painful problem is affecting their lives etc. Simply speak that back to them, you can even turn them into questions because that will result in them nodding their heads in agreement.

Osteobiz Tip #38

What are your patients complaining about?

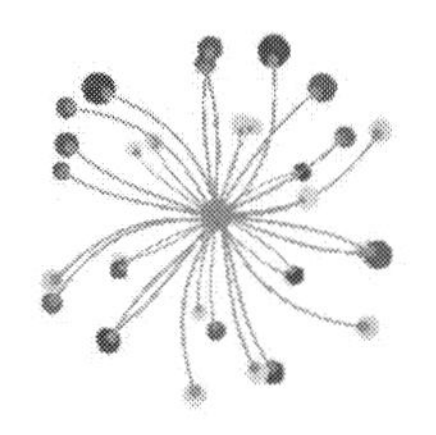

Go back to your marketing book and the notes you made; what are your patients complaining about? Write out some questions you can speak back to them.

For example, if your target market are sporty types, you could ask them:

- Are you struggling to get over injuries?
- Are your injuries seeing you side-lined to the benches at the weekend football match?
- Would you love to be fitter and move better?
- Did you know that Osteopathy can help you back to health?
- Did you know that Osteopathy can help you prepare for the skiing season?
- Did you know that Andy Murray, Chelsea FC Players and the Queen have regular Osteopathic treatments?

What Else Can I Do With These Questions?

Questions work so well because our brains automatically think about whether we already know something or whether it is new information which needs to be processed.

In your marketing, you can expand on these questions and turn them into attractive memes, matching the question with a striking image. You could also add a short statement such as *'Osteopaths love to treat pain and help you back to health'*.

Further, the question could be expanded to form the basis of a blog, video or newsletter.

Osteobiz Tip #39

Empty your head of all the questions you ever get asked, no matter how bizarre!

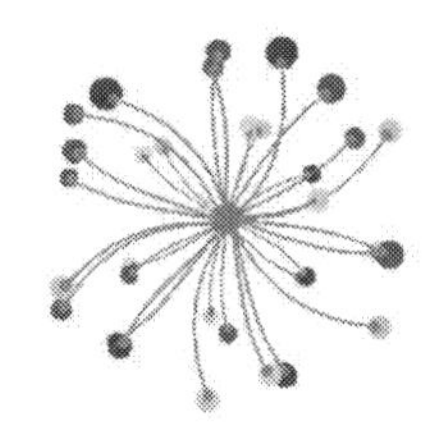

Note them down without filter, allow it to flow and write until you can think of no more!

What is calling out to you as a blog topic, meme or video demo?

It Feels Awkward To Ask For Testimonials, How Can I Do This Confidently?

(NOTE: Australian Regulations do not allow you to use Testimonials for promotional purposes. Check your own country's rules and abide by them.)

How does this sound?

- I want to build my practice, could you please give me a testimonial?
- I'm not busy enough, can you write me a testimonial please?
- When you get home, can you give me a Google review please? Thanks.

How is that feeling? Are you getting that icky feeling in your belly? Are you feeling compelled to help?

Let's take the emphasis off you and put it onto them:

- I would love to help more people like you. Could you please give me a few words about the difference Osteopathy has made to you?
- I'm passionate about helping more people like you out of pain and back to health. Is there one sentence which sums up your experience of Osteopathy?
- If someone else was suffering with the same problem as you, what would you say to them?

Osteobiz Tip #40

Testimonials demonstrate that other people value your skills.

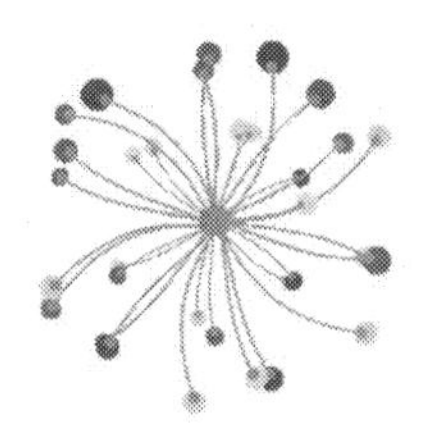

Go through your diary today; who would be a good person to ask? Who has seen a great improvement in their health and pain levels?

If they are seeing significant improvements since your treatment, they will surely be delighted to help others like themselves.

It is important to continuously encourage and inform your local community about the benefits of Osteopathic treatment. Testimonials ensure that the message is strong. They are some of the most powerful ways to ensure that you are helping people in pain to understand that they have options.

And as I say time and time again, if you're not getting that message out there in a variety of ways, how can you help them if they don't know you exist?

If they don't understand why they would invest in treatment then they will never ever book to see you.

How Can I Use A Case Study Without Breaching Confidentiality?

A case study can help to illustrate how you work and the general outcomes you achieve. I'm not a fan of listing conditions which the powers that be allow you to state that you treat. After all you are not trained to treat conditions per se.

Case studies are like a mini story and people love a story; especially one with a happy ending! So your case study can illustrate succinctly what a potential patient might expect.

If you create several case studies, you could use them as social media posts or turn them into a blog and even use as content in a newsletter too.

A case study should include how the patient felt before their first visit, what their problems stopped them from doing and how it generally affected their lives.

Following on from that, explain what treatment generally consisted of and the kind of advice you gave for self-care. An idea of the number of treatment sessions would help too.

The all-important outcomes will then help people to understand the benefits of Osteopathy in this type of case.

Osteobiz Tip #41

Amalgamate several typical patients and write a brief story about their return to health.

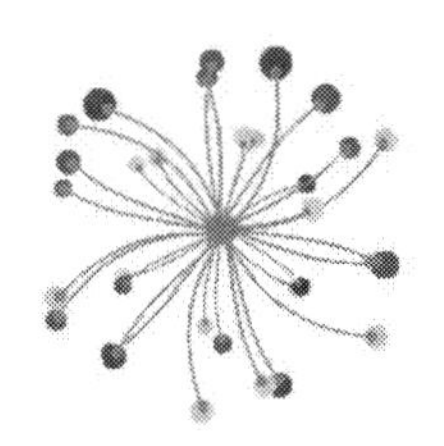

Take a broad overview of some of the cases you see. Could you do a generalised case study of the journey back to health that a typical patient takes?

If you have one or two patients who love your work and who have responded very well to treatment why not ask them if they would approve a case study with their name or a pseudonym?

Osteobiz Tip #42

Using photos on social media will help people to engage with your posts.

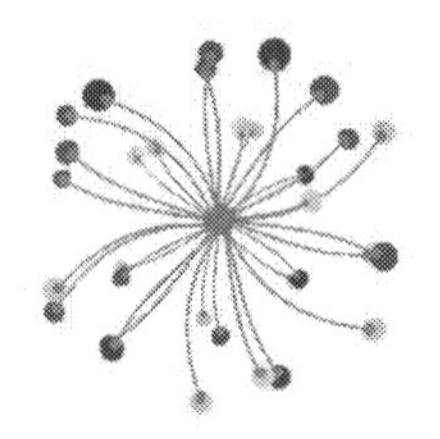

How Can I Use Photos In My Social Media Marketing?

It used to be that the privileged few had a decent camera with which to take photos. However, with the huge improvements in camera technology within mobile phones, we've all turned latter day David Baileys!

The benefits of using your own photos are many:

- There is no copyright to be concerned about.
- You have easy access to a range of photos.
- Online images tend to scream 'stock photo'.

Take it from me, most manual therapists are using the same dull old images of the same bodies with red heat marks on discs and joints!

Because we are very visual creatures and our social media newsfeeds are fast moving and colourful, images that you choose need to be poignant and appealing.

Images are also an important part of a blog, they help ground the topic, create curiosity and break up the text.

In-house leaflets will also benefit from customised and attractive images to illustrate the topic being discussed.

A well designed website will also need to include various persistent images to break up blocks of text and draw the eye to relevant sections.

For instance, an image of a baby will draw a mother's eye with ease to the paragraph of treatment for infants.

Osteobiz Tip #43

Text with eye-catching images on posts will encourage engagement.

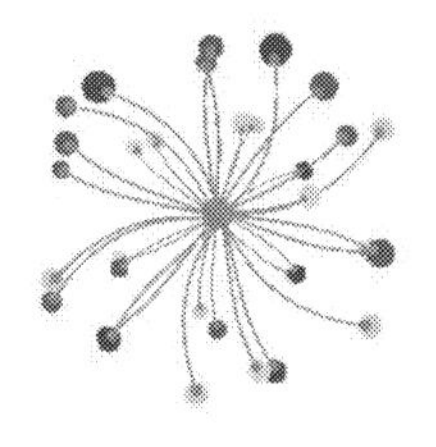

Huge blocks of text are a big turnoff to many who have little time but are hungry for information and solutions.

If you have patients who you know are keen to help you, maybe you could ask if they'd star in an image of treatment, even if they prefer to avoid their face being shown.

Alternatively, you could do the same exercise with colleagues or even family. I would strongly suggest that your face is visible though in as many as possible, this continues to allow local people to recognise you and trust you.

Should I Only Use Images of Treatment?

Social media is all about being social, as I've said before. So there are many types of images you could share in your marketing. Try out images of your treatment room, uncluttered waiting area, front door or even the parking area!

This all helps to make a person's first visit more familiar. It may also help the slightly nervous to feel reassured.

Osteobiz Tip #44

Creative use images other than the clinic and treatments can help to gain a huge amount of interaction.

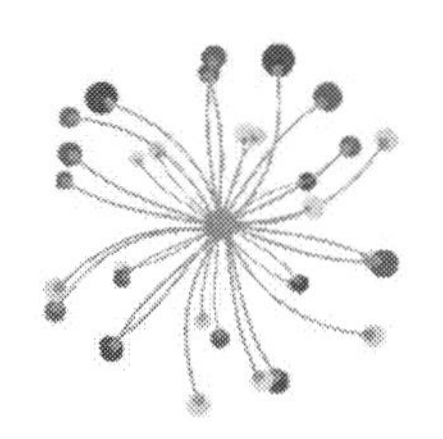

Why not go a step further and use images of local landmarks, frozen ponds in winter, pretty blossom in spring, the local bridal path in autumn and an epic summer scene at dusk?

These are all great talking points and are likely to get conversation going on your posts. A great picture is also likely to be shared, commented on, loved rather than liked and even have friends tagged in the comments to come and see it.

If you have pets you might even go one step further and include them looking playful, cheeky, or stealing your spot on your chair!

As crazy as it sounds, these kind of pictures are likely to give you way more exposure than a carefully constructed blog post.

Cute animals always attract attention, don't they? And if you're an animal Osteo, then you'll have a huge amount of opportunities to snap those grateful pets.

Are Videos A Good Idea?

The short answer is absolutely! For many years now I have been urging clients to use videos as a way to catapult their marketing results.

Sadly, on the whole, manual therapists are reluctant to step out of their comfort zone when it comes to videos.

What you do all day is demonstrate, explain and educate your patients. Your video is doing exactly the same but to a far wider audience, who've yet to discover you.

Remember that most people have no clue what goes on behind your front door! Show them, explain to them and help them to see you as the health expert that you are.

Osteobiz Tip #45

Videos need to account for a good 70% of the posts on your business page.

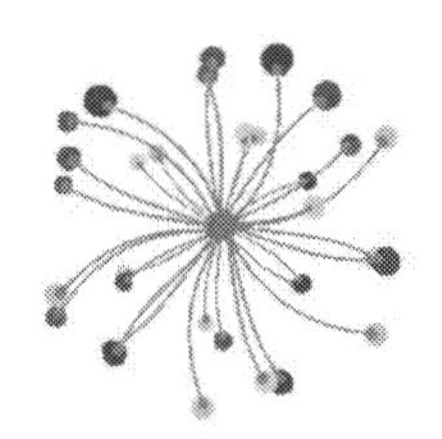

Get a colleague or friend to help you with filming. Videos need only be a couple of minutes long and demonstrate one idea or exercise.

For inspiration, think about the advice you give to your patients over and over again. Those will be great topics to begin with because clearly many people don't know what you know!

Remember the curse of knowledge and keep your language and explanations very concise, clear and certainly with no medical jargon; talking about MSK etc will not resonate with most people.

Here's my best tip to get over any nerves; you are not broadcasting to the entirety of Facebook or Instagram! You are only ever talking to just one person.

Doug may be sitting on the bus and idly looking through his Facebook feed for something to entertain him on the dull journey to work.

Or maybe Bob is mindlessly munching a dismal lunchtime cheese sandwich and searching for solutions for his computer-induced shoulder pain.

Ask yourself:

- What can you share with your perfect patients?
- What questions do they regularly ask?
- What misconceptions do they have?
- What advice would help them?
- What pertinent tips could you give them?

And there's no need for fancy equipment either. Simply begin with your phone, making sure that you are close enough for the volume to be good. Most people will forgive a less than perfect image but won't stick around if the sound quality is rubbish!

My final tip is to just be yourself; be confident, engaging and only refer to them in the singular. "Hi, guys," or, "Hello, everyone," is annoying when you are watching videos on your phone!

Is it Worth Doing a Facebook Live?

Facebook Lives have become very popular and are the very best way to get in front of your followers. Facebook is all about communication and entertainment and so their algorithm will put your Live out to way more people.

Lives can be longer than an ordinary video because the idea is to encourage people to join you in the moment and interact.

And if you're strategic about using this tool, you can step way ahead of your competitors! And yet again, it costs you nothing.

Osteobiz Tip #46

Deliver a live video from anywhere; your clinic, where you like to go running etc.

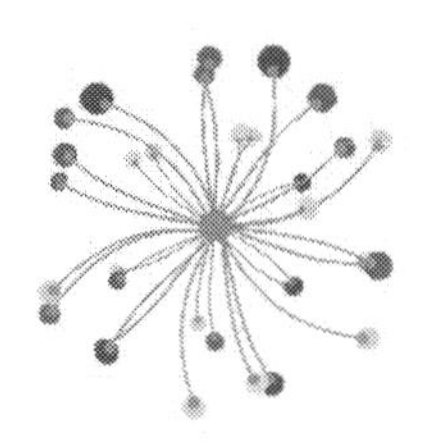

Choose a topic which you can discuss for about 10 minutes and make it interesting. Put a sticky note on the wall behind the camera or stick it on the front of your phone to guide you through your key points so that you don't waffle or lose your thread.

Discuss the topic, dispel any misconceptions and demonstrate with a volunteer patient if that illustrates your points better.

To choose the very best time to go on air, check out your Insights and see when most of your page followers are actively online.

Even better if you can create a regular slot and set up an event so that all of your followers will be notified.

Also, post a reminder on your page half an hour before to jog their memories too.

After recording the Live, you can click 'done' and it will post to your page for anyone else to watch later.

I promise you that if you do these regularly and market them well, you will get better reach to your page followers and in turn, that will translate into extra bookings.

Remember, nothing works like magic: marketing need to be ongoing and relentless. The world is a busy place and a message heard or seen once is unlikely to be retained consciously. You wouldn't believe how many new clients of mine say they've been following me and watching my stuff for a couple of years!

Imagine the different place they'd have been in by now if I'd got my hands on their Osteobiz back then!

What's the Point of Using Inspirational Quotes?

In a world where we are constantly bombarded by the negative news stories in the media, a little inspirational quote can lift the spirits. If you look swiftly through your personal newsfeed, you will see many that catch your eye.

Generally, the text is not too long , the quote is attributed, and it may or may not have a suitable image behind or next to the text.

It is important that you develop a style for your quotes, so that they're like a series. Even more critical is to use your correct branding fonts and colours (hex codes), so that your brand remains consistent and recognisable as you.

Remember that at least 80% of us are now using our social media on the small screens of our phones. It is vital that the meme you create is uncluttered and easy to read – no funny fonts which are too tricky for the eye to speedread.

Osteobiz Tip #47

Inspirational quotes can lift the spirits of your followers.

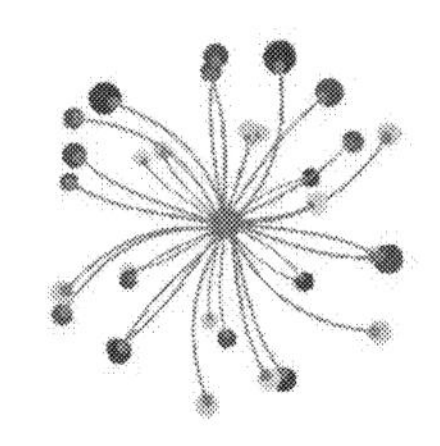

Screenshot the quote which makes you smile or nod in agreement or even chuckle! Use some of the Osteopathic greats to illustrate what Osteopathy stands for such as "To find health should be the object of the doctor. Anyone can find disease." AT Still.

Head to www.inspirationalquotes.com and scribble down the ones you believe are inspiring to your patients. For instance, if you specialise in treating the sporty, find the best quotes about tenacity and self-belief from Muhammed Ali, Usain Bolt and Serena Williams.

Set yourself a time limit and churn out as many as you can and schedule one to go out every Monday morning and watch their smiling emoticons pour in!

Osteobiz Tip #48

Memes are images with added text which convey a great message simply.

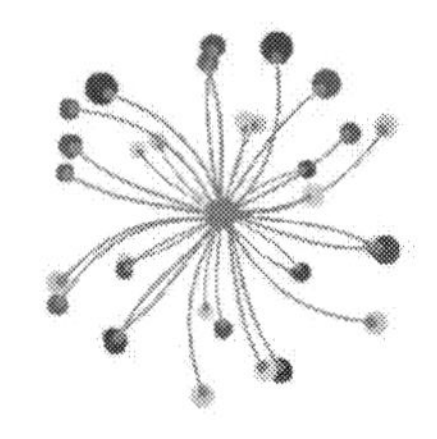

What On Earth Are Memes, And What Do I Do With Them?

Memes are the generic term for images with text on. You will see them appearing constantly in your social media newsfeeds.

As part of your array of content, they represent an important element. A meme allows you to convey a very strong message in an instant.

You can use any kind of pertinent image or even a plain background and add words on top to cement the idea or message.

There was a phase when many liked to use a sad face or a pained expression along with a dour message such as '*pain getting you down?*', or '*is old age a pain in the neck?*' etc. However, with Facebook being extremely keen to promote a positive experience for users, they're certainly not allowing those types of memes to be used in Facebook Ads for fear of offending. Facebook are highly sensitive to any references to mental health, weight or body shape etc.

With that in mind, I'm finding that rather than pressing 'pain points' too much, it's better to flip the coin and look at best outcomes, patient desires or aspirations, lifestyle or quality of life.

Try thinking about what your potential patient wishes for themselves. Jot down everything you've heard them say or know they would love.

For instance, if they're seniors, you could be posting memes of that age group doing the things they love again without pain.

Your text could say things like:

- Would you love to get back to your game of golf?
- Getting older doesn't have to mean getting old.
- Osteopathy keeps the spring in your step.

Remember strong messages create impact.

Don't be vanilla in a colourful world!

What Sort Of Tips And Advice Could I Give?

Social media is a great place to share nuggets of information. You can go back to your marketing book where you have feedback and insights and the misconceptions you've heard and turn them all around into bite-sized pieces of easily absorbed and digestible. Tips can be great for positioning yourself as an expert in health and wellbeing.

Look at your blogs and see if there are one-liners that would work well as a quick tip.

Osteobiz Tip #49

Memes make attention grabbing content for your audience.

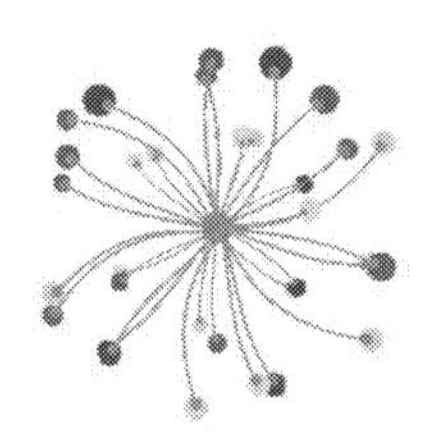

You could give tips on the correct use of hot and cold treatment for sporting injuries. You might want to give advice on getting the body moving first thing in the morning or even how to cool down after a bout of energetic gardening.

Once again, the most efficient way to do this is to grab a pen, your book and simply do a brain download and write everything down that flows. You can delete the ones you don't like afterwards but just allowing that free flow of thought gives you a huge amount of ideas to use as tips and advice.

Do You Think Infographics Are A Good Idea?

Personally, I don't have the kind of mind to create an infographic!

The whole idea of gathering statistics and showing them in different sections of the infographic leaves me cold!

However, as far as a tool for imparting statistics and information, they do deliver it in a succinct and direct manner.

Images and charts can be added to make it very visually appealing. Indeed, did you know that one of the best ways to make an infographic is by using PowerPoint?!

Osteobiz Tip #50

Share important statistics with an infographic.

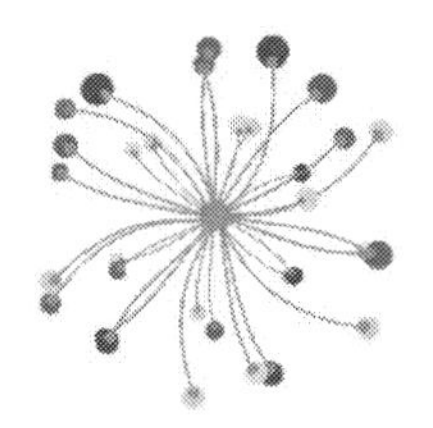

If your perfect patient would benefit from key information being delivered to them in a palatable form, then this may appeal.

I Don't Have Time To Post Stuff On Social Media – Shall I Get Someone Else To Do It?

This is a great question! I have to say, I have my reservations about using an external service to do your marketing for you.

My reasoning is this:

- You have strict regulations from your Governing Body about how you present yourself to the public. Therefore, it is difficult to relinquish that control to someone else without potentially being in breach of those regulations by proxy.
- Similarly, the Advertising Standards Agency (or your country's version of it) may receive complaints about the claims you're making in your marketing when you haven't been in control of that either.
- Osteopathy is a therapy which is taught differently in many different worldwide schools and colleges. Further, every Osteopath seems to interpret, hone and develop their skills differently. Hence, it is often the case that no two Osteopaths would express what they do in quite the same way. I liken this to

cooking – if you gave a Victoria Sponge recipe to 20 people, no 2 cakes would look or taste the same!

- Your message is quite complex in that most people don't understand what you do nor why they would visit you. I think that people outside of the profession who market plumbers and accountants would be less able to create effective marketing for you.
- The service you offer requires a good deal of trust on the part of a new patient. The way that you express yourself in your marketing helps people to get a sense of what you stand for. I feel strongly that it would be difficult to convey your personality, values and goals for your patients in a disjointed or arms-length way via an external party.

Osteobiz Tip #51

Schedule your social media posts and save time.

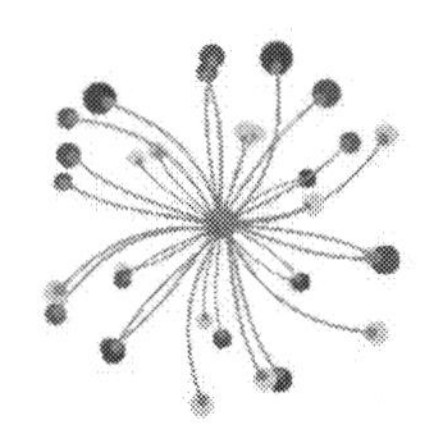

The solution to the conundrum of posting consistently is, I believe, to schedule some of your posts to social media. There are great tools on the market such as Buffer. Some are free for the basic level and others can be more like a library where they store all your content and simply repost over and over again.

On Facebook it is also possible to schedule your posts one by one, which is the most cost-effective. Once you've uploaded your piece of content, rather than click 'publish' you click the down arrow to the right of it and select schedule.

Once again, your insights will furnish you with information about the best times to post for you, but common sense helps too. For instance, you're more likely to catch your office workers online early morning whilst commuting rather than at 3pm when they're busy at their desks. Conversely, mothers may well be online at 3pm prior to collecting the kids from school but not early morning when they're trying to persuade the little darlings to go to school in uniform rather than PJs and slippers...

Ok, So I've Got All This Content Made Now, What's Next?

You've written killer blogs, you've made beautiful memes, churned out a shedload of tips, compiled a couple of epic infographics and you're sure to win an Oscar for your highly popular video series!

Now, my friend, you have created a whole library of content. Some is seasonal, some is topical, some is jolly well inspiring! But what now?

Here are the words you're gonna love...

Simply rinse and repeat!

Yes, you can now keep repeating and reposting all this lovely content. You have created a huge amount of evergreen social media posts which can continue to be uploaded multiple times.

Again, it's like driving a car. You really need to crank up through the gears, foot to the floor to get the wheels in motion. Once you've put in the effort, got the car zipping along in fifth gear and you're cruising, it's going to require much less effort from you to stay on track.

From now on, I'm pretty sure that you'll hear more misconceptions, misunderstandings etc. and you'll be straight onto the computer at your earliest opportunity to create another meme to address that, or whip up a quick blog to educate and inform more of your followers.

Over to you - it's time to implement!

This book was largely written whilst travelling through Bali, Australia and New Zealand whilst we were on a trip of a lifetime. I was very fortunate to meet with many Osteopaths on the way.

The final one I met in Auckland, just hours before I boarded a plane home. He was clearly a great thinker, as many of you are in your quest for greater understanding of the human condition, life, the universe and everything.

Beautiful metaphor after metaphor flowed from him, instantly giving me new understandings and raising new questions.

However, one comment struck me and totally resonated. It's what I am constantly trying to convey to new clients. But he said it better than I had ever managed before:

"*Challenge creates change.*"

So, in the challenge of doing something new to solve a problem, you disrupt the norm and change happens.

As I get older, I hear more and more people bemoaning change. "Oh, it's not like it used to be..." they whinge.

I never understand why anyone wants everything to stay the same. The Old Boy decries the fact that the John Lewis Partnership, who he worked for for over 30 years, has changed.

But, of course, if it had stayed the same as it was 30 years ago, the rest of the world would have moved on and ultimately it would have likely vegetated and eventually collapsed as so many other multiples have; like our dearest beloved Woolworths!

I believe that it is vital to embrace change. Rather than the negative commentaries which emanate from the media, often shaping our worldview, I think that if we instead look for opportunities, options and openings we can find the new path, move forwards and develop ourselves, our businesses, and our gifts.

Many Osteopaths come to me with dramatically reducing bookings. They can't fathom how they used to be really booked up but now are not.

Often, they will resort to trying the same marketing tactics over and again but still no change!

Now you know why:

"*Challenge creates change.*"

So, in the challenge of manifesting new patients, more bookings and improved income, the required changes will transpire.

And that's why an annual review of your business is paramount. Testing what's working, what's not and what changes need to be made to keep the business moving forward. This is especially true in such a period of monumental technological change as we are experiencing now.

Much like sailing a boat, the skipper must constantly correct his course. If he makes no change, he will surely run aground or at best end up in a place that he hadn't planned to.

This book is just a start to getting you on the road to marketing yourself with confidence. The critical steps to take now are to market yourself consistently and persistently. And with that constant momentum, you'll see growth in your business.

However, if you feel you need a guiding hand and some accountability to help you to grow a thriving practice and health hub for your community, then book yourself in for a free consultation.

https://osteobiz.as.me/consultation

Book in and find out how Osteopaths around the world are rapidly growing patient numbers on the year long Osteobiz Mastermind programme.

Since Osteopath Jos Drew joined me at Osteobiz HQ in November 2018, we've been able to further increase the depth of support and mentoring to our clients. And their results demonstrate that the methods we have devised and honed are making all the difference.

Many clients typically report shifting from a handful of patients per week to massively increased bookings with others saying that they simply feel more confident in running their business. And these are outcomes that we're very proud to be a part of. Every day we're helping more people around the world, who are in pain, to find their local Osteopath. And that's the bigger picture - or you might say a BHAG!

Now back to Toby!

Frankly, we had a few tough years and he struggled massively at times. In 2008, when we returned to the UK, Toby's Cardiologists had hoped that he might benefit from a few months' growth to enable him to receive a slightly larger heart than that of a child.

But the miracle that ensued was as much a surprise to the doctors as it was to us.

And I strongly believe that regular osteopathic treatments were the defining component in him managing to get through senior school and secure excellent sixth form qualifications in performing arts, without needing a new heart.

In September 2013, just as I was creating the foundations of Osteobiz, the (third time lucky) call came for Toby's transplant. It was with great sadness that we accepted the healthy heart of someone who had tragically died too young. We are forever grateful to that anonymous family and we always think of their loss in September and at Christmas.

It was now 5 whole years since our hasty return from Athens and Toby was a tall and lanky 17 year old. The Consultants at Great Ormond Street Hospital were amazed at his energy, given the severe chemotherapy induced cardiomyopathy he had been coping with.

Toby had exceeded all our expectations by managing to cycle energetically everywhere, study and party with just a few meds and a regular 'top up' of osteopathy, which always seemed to magically re-energise him.

He's since powered into his early twenties and now works in a demanding job in admin and accounts.

You might say that, after 20 years of stressful shenanigans, it's 'my time' now. And so every day I am engrossed in continuing to innovate and build a successful global business for promoting Osteopathy and focus on my greater mission to help more people in the world to find this efficient and sometimes life-changing treatment.

Makes me kind of glad too that my reed basket empire and life enhancing elixir never quite took off back in the 1970s.

Because, after motherhood, my work in the osteopathic world is most definitely my calling in life.

Connect with Gilly

https://www.osteobiz.com/

Online social media workshop:

http://bit.ly/osteobizws

Social media:

https://www.facebook.com/Osteobiz/

https://www.instagram.com/gillywoodhouse/

https://twitter.com/GillyWoodhouse

https://www.linkedin.com/in/gillywoodhouse/

Printed in Great
Britain
by Amazon